DADI MA
फलों KE
The Healing
FRUITS

Nita Mehta

B.Sc. (Home Science), M.Sc. (Food and Nutrition), Gold Medalist

Co-author
Harveen Choudhary

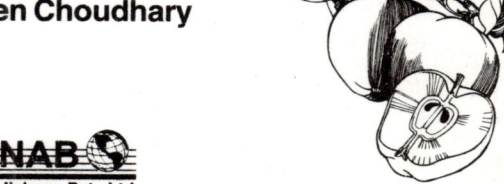

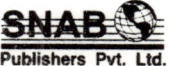

SNAB
Publishers Pvt. Ltd.

DADI MAA KE फलों KE NUSKHE

© Copyright 2001-2002 **SNAB** Publishers Pvt. Ltd.

WORLD RIGHTS RESERVED. The contents—all recipes, photographs and drawings are original and copyrighted. No portion of this book shall be reproduced, stored in a retrieval system or transmitted by any means, electronic, mechanical, photocopying, recording or otherwise, without the written permission of the publishers.

While every precaution is taken in the preparation of this book, the publisher and the author assume no responsibility for errors or omissions. Neither is any liability assumed for damages resulting from the use of information contained herein.

TRADEMARKS ACKNOWLEDGED. Trademarks used, if any, are acknowledged as trademarks of their respective owners. These are used as reference only and no trademark infringement is intended upon.

2nd Print 2002
ISBN 81-7869-001-2

Illustrations and Photography: **SNAB**

Layout and laser typesetting :

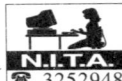

National Information Technology Academy
3A/3, Asaf Ali Road
New Delhi-110002
☎ 3252948

Published by :
SNAB Publishers Pvt. Ltd.
3A/3 Asaf Ali Road,
New Delhi-110002
Tel: 3252948, 3250091

Editorial and Marketing office:
E-348, Greater Kailash-II, N.Delhi-48
Fax: 91-11-6235218 Tel: 91-11-6214011, 6238727
E-Mail: nitamehta@email.com
snab@snabindia.com
Website: http://www.nitamehta.com
Website: http://www.snabindia.com

Distributed by :
THE VARIETY BOOK DEPOT
A.V.G. Bhavan, M 3 Con Circus,
New Delhi - 110 001
Tel : 3327175, 3322567; Fax : 3714335

Printed by :
THOMSON PRESS (INDIA) LTD.

Rs. 69/-

Introduction

Fruits have great therapeutic value or healing power to cure innumerable diseases. About 2,500 years ago Hippocrates - the father of medicine, said, **"Not the Doctor, but Nature Heals"**.

Fruits increase vitality, strengthen the immune system, regulate weight and slow down the ageing process because they are packed with vitamins and minerals and are low in fats. They also boost energy levels and help to detoxify the body. Fruits contain enzymes which are needed to digest food, absorb nutrients effectively, metabolise fats and destroy toxins. In short, these are essential for the body to perform it's routine functions effectively and protect you from illnesses.

No amount of vitamin pills can give a glow to your skin if the internal organs are not functioning properly. Heavily cooked and processed foods are "dead foods" and it is only "living foods" like fruits which will nourish the body. Thus fruits are rightfully called the **Nectar of Life!**

Nita Mehta

Contents

Natural Benefits and Healing Properties of Fruits

- INTRODUCTION 3
- How and when to eat fruits 5
- Fruits cleanse the body of toxic wastes 6
- Apricot (*Khumani*) 8
- Apple (*Seb*) 11
- Almond (*Badaam*) 15
- Avocado (*Makhanphal*) 21
- Banana (*Kela*) 23
- Coconut (*Nariyal*) 29
- Date (*Khajoor*) 34
- Fig (*Anjeer*) 38
- Grapefruit (*Chakotra*) 42
- Grape (*Angoor*) 46
- Guava (*Amrood*) 51
- Indian Gooseberry (*Amla*) 54
- Jambul Fruit (*Jamun*) 59
- Musk Melon (*Kharbooja*) 61
- Lemon (*Niboo*) 63
- Mango (*Aam*) 69
- Mulberry (*Shahtoot*) 74
- Orange (*Santra*) 75
- Papaya (*Papita*) 79
- Pineapple (*Ananas*) 83
- Pomegranate (*Anar*) 85
- Plums (*Aloo Bukhara*) 88
- Peaches (*Aadu*) 89
- Strawberries 90
- Sweet Lime (*Mosambi*) 91
- Watermelon (*Tarbuz*) 93
- Walnut (*Akhrot*) 97

How & When To Eat Fruits
Do Not End The Meal With a Fruit

Fruit should never be taken with or immediately following a meal. It is essential that when you eat fruit, it is taken on an empty stomach.

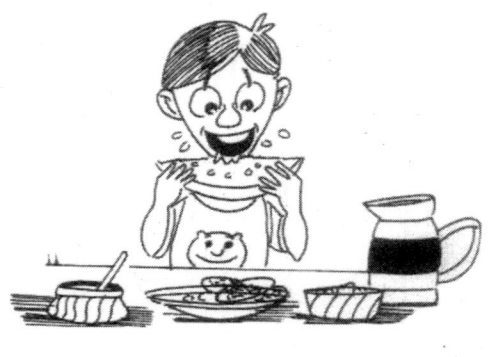

Fruit does not digest in the stomach, unlike other foods. Fruits are predigested. All fruits (with the exception of bananas, dates and dried fruit, which stay in the stomach a bit longer) are in the stomach only for a very short time. On the other hand, other foods spend 1-1½ hours in the stomach to get digested. Fruits pass through the stomach in 20-30 minutes as if they were going through a tunnel. They breakdown and release their supercharged, life giving nutrients in the intestine. But if fruits are taken with other foods, they get locked in the stomach with other foods where they ferment. For example, water melon will never create gas when taken the first thing in the morning, but if it is taken after a meal, it may give you a lot of discomfort.

Fruits Cleanse the Body of Toxic Wastes
Start The Day With Fruit

Eating fruit correctly plays a major role in cleansing the body of toxic wastes. This is because fruits contain enzymes which destroy toxins.

Start the day with a fruit, by taking fruit on an empty stomach. It is best to eat fruit in the morning and about 20 minutes before the other breakfast foods (cereals, breads, milk, tea etc.) so that by the time you eat the other foods, the fruit has already left the stomach and passed on to the intestine for absorption of important nutrients.

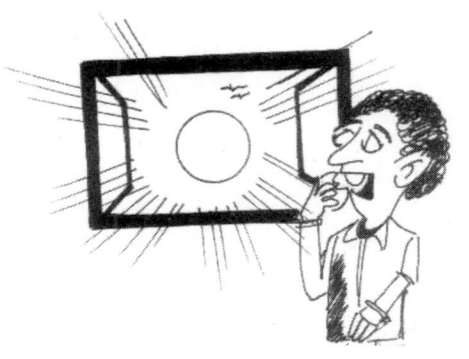

A toxic acid system can be recognized by bloating, excess weight, celluloid, nervous outbursts, greying hair, balding, dark circles under the eyes and premature lines in the face. When you have totally mastered the principle of correct fruit consumption, you have tuned into nature's secrets of good health, longevity, beauty and normal weight.

Apricot (*Khumani*)

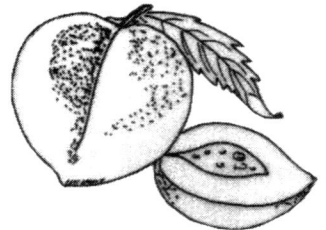

Apricot is also called the apple of gold because in olden days the Chinese used to make a famous medicine known as apricot gold from kernels of apricot. This medicine was reputed to have the power to prolong life to a great extent.

Apricot is considered an excellent food remedy due to its high **iron** content. There is a small amount of copper also present and its presence makes the iron easily available to our bodies.

The apricot is yellowish in colour and is either round or oblong with a single nut (seed) in it. The ripe fruit is sweetish being rich in natural sugars, **Vitamin A and Vitamin C.** It is also a good source of **vitamin B complex.** The nut is rich in **protein and oil.** The oil is somewhat like almond oil and is widely used for many ailments.

NATURAL HEALING THROUGH APRICOTS

- **Anaemia:** Apricots being high in iron content are beneficial in the treatment of anaemia. The small amount of copper present in apricots helps in quick absorption of iron by our bodies. Thus the production of haemoglobin can be greatly increased thereby overcoming anaemia by eating apricots liberally.
- **Constipation:** Apricots have a high protein and cellulose (fibre) content. The cellulose is not easily digested and thus forms bulk which stimulates bowel movement. Hence consumption of 7-8 apricots daily acts as a mild laxative providing relief from constipation.
- **Fevers:** Ripe apricots or their juice is very beneficial in fevers as it is very cooling and a thirst quencher. In addition, it acts like a tonic by supplying various minerals and vitamins. The apricot pieces and its juice can be had plain or for better results, it can be mixed with some honey.

APRICOTS FOR BEAUTY

Apricot has nourishing and firming qualities. It therefore nourishes, rejuvenates and tightens your skin. It also helps in lightening stretch marks and smoothening wrinkles. Grate a ripe apricot and apply the pulp or juice on the face and neck or simply take an apricot slice and rub it all over. Leave for 20 minutes before washing off. It is good for all types of skins. Apricot is a popular ingredient in many beauty/cosmetic preparations such as face scrubs, masks etc.

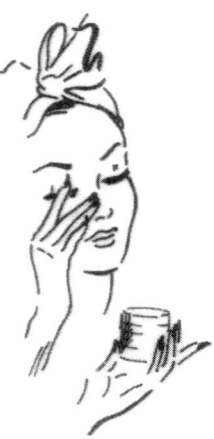

MORE ABOUT APRICOTS

Apricots are eaten fresh or as a dry fruit. Apricots are used to prepare exotic desserts and sauces. They are also used to make preserves like - jams, jelly and marmalade. Its seed or nut is used to make oil which is very useful in making cosmetics.

Apple (*Seb*)

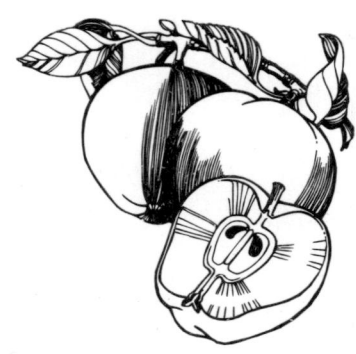

Everyone of us is familiar with the saying, "An apple a day keeps the doctor away." This is said keeping in mind the various medicinal uses, nourishing and health promoting properties of the apple.

The **skin** of the apple should not be discarded as the skin and the flesh just below it contain **more vitamin C** than the inner flesh. The skin also contains **5 times more vitamin A** than the inner flesh.

They are highly nutritive containing a good amount of **iron, calcium, arsenic, phosphorus and vitamin A.** Small amounts of **vitamin E and B complex** are also present.

Natural Healing Through Apples

- **Heart disease:** Apples are high in potassium and phosphorus content and very low (practically nil) in sodium. This fact is of great advantage in heart diseases. Consuming apples with honey proves to be an effective food remedy in heart problems.
- **High Blood Pressure:** People suffering from high B.P are advised to go on an apple diet for a few days. This is highly beneficial as it contains almost no sodium. Its diuretic effect increases the secretion of urine, bringing down the blood pressure. Apples also lower the sodium content in the tissues. They are rich in potassium and also benefit the kidneys.
- **Arthritis and Gout:** Apples are very effective in the treatment of gout and arthritis. These conditions are caused by the accumulation of uric acid. The malic acid present in apples neutralises this uric acid and hence gives relief to the patients.
- **Anaemia:** Apples are very rich in iron. They are therefore a good food remedy for treating anaemia. The apples can be eaten raw or

consumed in the juice form. However a large amount of apples approximately one kg daily, should be consumed for beneficial results.

- **Cough:** The high pectin content of apples relieves cough and helps in eliminating toxins from the body. A minimum of 300-350 gms of apples or their juice should be consumed daily for 8-10 days for beneficial results.
- **Constipation and Diarrhoea:** Apples are good, both for constipation and diarrhoea. Uncooked or raw apples, the apples in their natural state, are good for diarrhoea. For constipation, cooked or baked apples are good as the cooking process softens the cellulose and provides bulk to the faeces.
- **Eye problems:** Boil apple peel with water for a few minutes. Strain and sweeten with honey. Drink this or use it as an eye wash (for eye wash, honey can be omitted) for beneficial results in all eye problems.
- **Nerve Tonic:** Apple with milk and honey can be taken in the form of a milk-shake. It acts as a nerve tonic recharging the nerves with new life and energy.

- **Protector of teeth:** The acid content of apples has an antiseptic influence and mouth cleaning property equal to no other fruit. When apples are eaten by chewing and masticating them, they exert an antiseptic influence on the germs present in the mouth thus preventing these germs to produce any harmful effects. The apple can therefore be considered a natural mouth cleanser and protector of teeth.

APPLES FOR BEAUTY

Mashed apple used as a face pack delays the onset of wrinkles.

Rubbing a slice of apple on your teeth is also helpful in getting your teeth sparkling white.

MORE ABOUT APPLES

Apples are used in the preparation of salads, desserts, jams, jelly and vinegar. It can also be baked or cooked. **Raw** apples consumed on an empty stomach may give indigestion. Apples should be avoided in the case of a sore throat.

Almond (*Badaam*)

Almond is a special nut which is highly nutritious and has very positive qualities. It is called a *brain and body* tonic as it provides us with nearly all the elements that we need for positive health building. It also serves as a valuable food remedy for several common ailments.

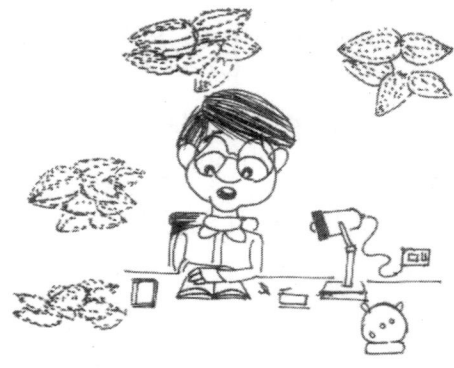

There are two varieties of almonds - sweet and bitter. Here we refer to the sweet almond with which we are all familiar. The bitter variety is generally not consumed as it contains a poisonous substance and is commercially used for extracting oil and in the manufacture of perfumes and cosmetics.

Almond contains approximately **20% protein** - a protein which can be very easily digested. Almonds though rich in fat, provide one of the most beneficial kinds of **fat,** which is **unsaturated**. Thus it helps in **lowering serum cholesterol levels.**

NATURAL HEALING THROUGH ALMONDS

- **Brain tonic:** Our grandmothers always said, "Oh! You are studying so hard, you must have 5 or 7 soaked almonds everyday to sharpen and feed your brain." It has been an age old saying that almonds are an excellent brain tonic. The recommended method is to soak 5 or 7 almonds overnight in water. Next morning remove the skin and eat the almonds with a cup of milk.
- **Cancer:** Almonds have a rich composition and favourable influence on the calcium balance and the defence mechanism of our bodies. They are therefore highly recommended for consumption in the diet of a cancer patient.
- **Constipation:** Almonds being laxative in nature are very beneficial

for constipation. Soak 3-4 almonds with 2-3 dried figs (*anjeer*) in a cup of water in the morning. At night remove the skin of almonds and grind both almonds and figs to a paste. Add little honey and have this at bedtime for a few days, to facilitate clear motions next morning.

- Simply eat 10-15 almonds at bed time and you will find that your bowels move very well the next morning.
- **Early stages of Cataract:** Soak 10-12 almonds in a cup of water overnight. Next morning remove skin and grind the almonds with 10-12 peppercorns (*saboot kaali mirch*) to a paste. Add a cup of water and honey or sugar to taste. Drink once daily. Continue for a few weeks. This will strengthen the eyes to regain their normal conditions and also cure hoarseness of the throat.
- **Anaemia:** Almonds contain copper which along with iron and vitamins acts as a catalyst in the synthesis of blood haemoglobin. Hence consumption of almonds is a sure shot remedy for anaemia.
- **Kidney and liver disorders:** People suffering from these disorders benefit greatly by including almonds in their daily diets.

- **Milk for Babies:** The babies or children who have an allergy to milk can be fed almond milk. The protein present in almonds makes it an excellent supplement for milk.
- **Tonic:** Almonds are an energy giving and high-calorie value food. They therefore serve as a tonic for children and elders. For better assimilation in our systems almonds should be consumed in combination with peppercorns (*saboot kali mirch*), poppy seeds (*khuskhus*) and green cardamoms (*illaichi*). *Shardai*, the popular almond drink is made by combining almonds with all these ingredients.
- **Sexual weakness:** Almonds are basically an energy giving and health building food. It is therefore very beneficial in sexual weakness as its consumption imparts strength. It also gives strength in nervous weakness and helps in sharpening the brain.

ALMONDS FOR BEAUTY

Almonds are said to render beauty. Hence their intake or external application or the massage with its oil greatly enhances the complexion and brings a glow to the person's face.

Mix together 1 teaspoon almond oil with ½ teaspoon fresh lemon juice. Apply under eyes (on the dark circles) and leave for 20-25 minutes. Done regularly the dark circles will begin to fade.

Mix equal amounts of almond oil (*badaam rogan*) with honey. Apply on face regularly. Keep for 10-15 minutes before washing off.

Massage face and neck with almond oil regularly to prevent wrinkles. This is recommended for dry skin only. People with oily skin should not do this or they might break out in pimples.

For a very dry skin, mix together 1 teaspoon almond oil and 1 teaspoon olive oil. Apply on the face and neck. You can also massage for a few minutes. Then leave it on for 15-20 minutes before washing off. This treatment should be done at least 2-3 times a day and increased if your skin is still feeling dry.

More About Almonds

Almonds are eaten as a dry fruit. They are used in salads, desserts, soup and sherbet. The oil extracted from almonds finds a lot of use in cosmetics and pharmaceutical industries.

As the almonds are heaty they should be drowned in water i.e. soaked overnight, skin discarded and then consumed during summers. However eating them with skin during winter will bring warmth to the body.

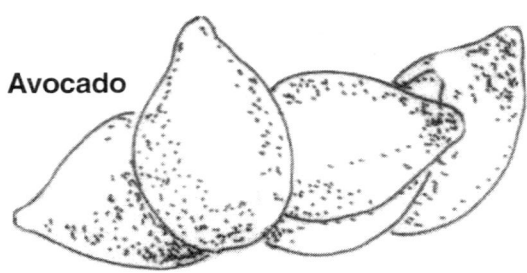
Avocado

Avocado (*Makhanphal*)

Avocado contains more fat than any other fruit except olives. It also contains **vitamin A, calcium, phosphorus, Iron** and some amount of **vitamin E**.

Avocado is not a highly cultivated plant. There are varieties of Avocado, ranging in size from small to large, pear-shaped to round, smooth skinned or rippled, green to almost black in colour. There is only one large seed inside which is surrounded by a pale yellow buttery pulp and a hard skin.

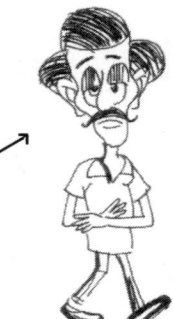

- **Malnutrition:** It is effective in cases of malnutrition and has the reputation of being an excellent tissue builder.
- **Digestive complaints:** Its blandness makes it an ideal food for people suffering from chronic digestive troubles. It has a soothing effect on the

digestive tract and the vitamins present in it help in the build up and repair of the inflamed tract.
- **Dysentery and Diarrhoea:** The seed of avocado is roasted and ground. 2 teaspoon of this powder mixed with a cup of lukewarm water, given 1-2 times a day helps to cure diarrhoea and dysentery.

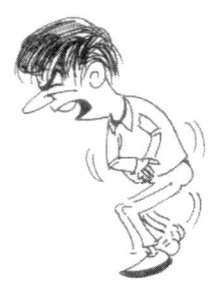

AVOCADO FOR BEAUTY

Mash the pulp of avocado well and mix with some curd. Apply on the face to prevent the ageing effect and on the hair for a natural hair conditioner to revitalize dull hair. An avocado paste applied on hands, soothes and softens them.

MORE ABOUT AVOCADO

Avocado is generally used in salads and in making dips. Guacamole, the famous Mexican dip is prepared from avocados.

Avocados turn sour on cooking, so it is advisable to use them raw.

Banana (*Kela*)

Banana is one of the oldest, most cultivated and easily available fruit. It comes with an easily removable peel and at a very reasonable price. Although low in price its importance is truly worth noting. The mature fruit has different sizes and colours. They may vary in size from 3" to 8" and in colour from green, yellow to reddish. The raw banana is also used as a vegetable.

The banana is of great nutritional value. It is **low in sodium and rich in potassium, calcium** and **iron**. It has a good sodium-potassium balance. It is a good source of calories and as it contains a large amount of easily assimilable sugar, it provides us with quick recovery from fatigue. The banana along with milk is called an almost complete balanced diet, because banana and milk supplement each other ideally.

Natural Healing Through Bananas

- **Depression:** Banana contains *serotonin*, a neurotransmitter that makes nerve contact possible. Lack of serotonin in the brain can result in depression and suicidal tendencies. Thus banana is a very important fruit and must be included in the daily diet of people suffering from depression.
- **Allergies:** Banana is useful for a lot of people who suffer from allergies, whether in the form of asthma or skin rash or stomach upsets. However a few (a minority) people may be allergic to bananas and after testing they should avoid it.
- **Anaemia:** It is a special food for the anaemic. As it is rich in iron it stimulates the production of haemoglobin in the blood. It is also helpful in cases of weakness and general loss of strength.

- Another remedy for anaemia is to mix 1 tablespoon of amla juice with one ripe banana. Mash well and have 2-3 times a day for a few days.
- A ripe banana mashed with 1 tablespoon of honey is also very beneficial in anaemia.

- **Arthritis and gout:** A diet of only bananas for 3-4 days is beneficial in the case of arthritis and gout. The patient can have 8-9 bananas every day during this time.
- **Burns and wounds:** Mash a ripe banana well so as to form a smooth paste. Apply on wounds and burns and tie a cloth bandage on it for immediate relief. Banana leaves are also said to form a cool dressing for blisters and inflammation.
- **Cancer:** Banana possesses an excellent potassium-sodium balance (proportion) and that is very important in the diet of a cancer patient.
- **Constipation:** Bananas are unique in that they are useful in both constipation as well as diarrhoea. They are rich in pectin which absorbs water thus forming bulk and relieving constipation. Therefore for proper bowel movement inclusion of 2-3 bananas in your daily diet

is a must for people suffering from constipation.

- **Diarrhoea:** To cure diarrhoea mash a ripe banana with a pinch of salt and 1 tablespoon tamarind pulp and have it at least 2 times daily for a few days.
- **Diabetes:** The unripe banana is very beneficial when included in a diabetics' diet.
- **Dysentery:** The combination of ripe banana, salt and tamarind pulp is very effective in dysentery. Bananas are also useful in dysentery of children. Only make sure that they are nice and ripe and mash them well into a pulp before giving to the child.
- **Piles:** As bananas relieve constipation they are also useful in the treatment of piles. Take a ripe banana, cut into small pieces or grate it. Boil it well with a cup of milk. Have this 2-3 times daily.
- **Ulcers:** Bananas have miraculous anti-ulcer properties. Green bananas are more potent than ripe bananas. Include raw bananas in your diet but take care to cook them well. Banana is said to contain an

unidentified compound called Vitamin U which is said to be an enemy of ulcer. It acts upon the lining of the stomach and neutralises the over acidity of the acid in the stomach and thus reduces irritation.

BANANAS FOR BEAUTY

Mash a ripe banana and mix some rose water to it. Used regularly as a face mask delays wrinkles.

Mash one ripe banana well. Add equal amounts of warm olive oil or coconut oil. Use as a face pack. It nourishes and moisturises your skin thoroughly.

MORE ABOUT BANANAS

Ripe bananas are eaten as a fruit for breakfast or as a dessert. The poor labourers have a few bananas with their lunch as it gives strength and energy. Bananas can also be used in salads and fruit chat.

Unripe bananas are cooked and eaten as a vegetable specially during fasts. Banana wafers made from unripe bananas are very popular. The flour made from unripe bananas is very rich in minerals and being easily digestible is an ideal food for *invalids and infants*.

Eating bananas in excess causes gas. People suffering from kidney failure should not eat bananas as it has a high percentage of potassium.

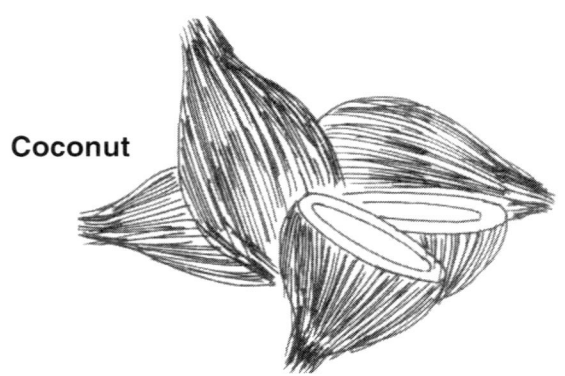

Coconut

Coconut (*Nariyal*)

Coconut is a sacred fruit and is used in all religious festivals. It is considered a near perfect diet or a **wonder food** as it contains almost all the essential nutrients required by the human body. In traditional households an **expectant mother** is encouraged to consume coconut as it provides all the essential vitamins, minerals and enzymes required by the growing foetus.

The coconut fruit is three angled and one seeded. It is surrounded by fibres and a hard shell with three markings on one side called the eyes. Inside is a white edible kernel which we commonly know as coconut. There is a central hollow cavity containing water.

The mature coconut is very rich in oil, high quality proteins, potassium, sodium, magnesium and sulphur. It also has a fair amount of niacin. The young coconut or the young green coconut is richer in enzymes and minerals than the mature one. It's water has cleansing properties, is bacteria free, cool, nourishing and diuretic. The water of one young coconut has enough **vitamin C** to meet our daily requirement. It is also a rich source of other vitamins from group **B**. Coconut is used in all stages of maturity.

NATURAL HEALING THROUGH COCONUTS

- **Acidity:** Drinking water of young tender coconut overcomes acidity. Drink a glass of coconut water every few (2-3) hours for a few days in case of very severe acidity.
- **Cancer:** Of all the foodstuffs, coconut contains the largest amount of *selenium*, which is an important part of an enzyme present in the human body. This enzyme is very important in the metabolic process of poly unsaturated fatty acids and prevents the development of free radicals. Hence, coconut consumption is very beneficial in cases of cancer.

- **Cholera:** Coconut water is indisputable in cholera. In cases of cholera the patient on account of loose motions and vomiting loses a lot of body fluids and this can lead to dehydration. Coconut water, being rich in potassium and mineral, when given to cholera patients helps prevent dehydration and also corrects the electrolyte balance of the body. In addition as the water is antibacterial, it helps in expelling the cholera germs from the intestines.
- **Dry Cough:** An effective remedy for dry cough and throat irritation is made from coconut milk. Take some freshly extracted coconut milk and mix with 1 tablespoon of poppy seeds (*khus khus*) and honey. Have 1 tablespoon of this mixture every night for a few days.
- **Mouth Ulcer:** Mixing some coconut milk with honey and massaging the affected area a few times a day gives relief.
- **Pain in Hips:** Extract some coconut milk from a ripe coconut. Cook some fenugreek (*methi*) leaves in it. Add an egg to it. Eat this 2-3 times a day for relief from pain in the hips.
- **Piles:** Pulp of tender coconut is used for piles and the oil from the nut when externally applied controls the pain due to piles.

- **Stomach Ulcers:** Drinking coconut water of young green coconut or milk extracted from mature coconut gives quick relief.
- **Urinary Trouble:** Coconut water is a natural diuretic. Water of ripe coconut promotes flow of urine. Hence it is very useful in urinary troubles, high B.P. and cases of kidney stones. It also strengthens the heart and vitalizes the nerves and the digestive system as it is very rich in vitamin B.
- **Worms in the Intestine:** Kernel of a ripe coconut is excellent for the expulsion of worms particularly tapeworm. Grate the coconut and have 2 tablespoon of this followed by a dose of castor oil after 2-3 hours. Repeat this everyday till the worms have been expelled.

Coconuts For Beauty

Apply coconut water (from fresh tender coconut) on face and neck. Rinse off with water after 20 minutes. Coconut water makes all marks disappear, even marks left by chicken pox (provided they are not very old) within a short time.

For thick, lustrous hair, heat some coconut oil. Massage well into scalp. Leave overnight. Shampoo next day. Coconut oil nourishes the scalp and also promotes hair growth. This should be done at least once a week.

More About Coconut

The milk of fresh coconut is a valuable food for children suffering from malnutrition and other nutritional deficiencies. To take out coconut milk, grate the coconut and add 2 cups of hot water to it. Keep aside for 30 minutes and then blend in a blender. Strain through a muslin cloth to get coconut milk. Green coconut water is used as a drink. It is a great thirst quencher, cool and highly nutritious. Kernel of ripe coconut is used in salads, cooking and the milk extracted from coconut occupies a high position in some cuisines such as Goan and Thai.

Too much consumption of mature coconut will add to weight gain as it is a very fatty food. Excessive use of water of tender coconut may cause difficult or painful urination.

Note: Desiccated coconut is not suitable for medicinal purposes.

Date (*Khajoor*)

Date is called the all purpose fruit. It is highly nutritive and thus of great importance. As its original home is said to be either the Persian Gulf or Mesopotamia, the date is also called the bread of the Sahara. However its use and cultivation has become very widespread now.

There are 2 main types of dates - fresh dates (*khajoor*) and dry dates (*chhuara*). The fresh dates are soft where as the dry dates are hard. Soft dates are quite moist and contain 60% sugar in the form of glucose and fructose where as in the dry dates the sugar content is between 65-70%. The tree-ripe date is a delicious fruit but it undergoes fermentation very fast, so it has to be dried in the sun. Their main advantage is that they can be stored for a long time and are undamaged by transportation. Apart from natural sugars, dates are fairly rich in **nicotinic acid, iron, potassium and calcium.** They also contain protein, a small amount of fat, fibre, vitamin A, B, B2 and also traces of magnesium, sulphur and copper.

NATURAL HEALING THROUGH DATES

- **Weak Heart:** A weak heart benefits tremendously by the consumption of dates. Soak a few dates in water overnight. Crush them the next morning in the same water (remove seeds) and drink it at least 2-3 times a week for strengthening a weak heart.

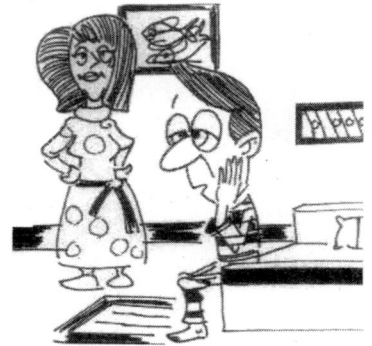

- **Sexual Weakness:** As dates are great energy givers they are helpful in cases of sexual weakness. Soak a handful of dates in goat's milk overnight. Remove seed and grind them the next morning. Add a pinch of cardamom (*chhoti illaichi*) powder and honey to taste. Drink it. This acts as a tonic and is very helpful in overcoming sexual weakness.

- **Teething problems in children:** Children during teething normally suffer from diarrhoea or dysentery. 1 teaspoon of date paste prepared with honey given 2-3 times a day is very beneficial in overcoming this problem.
- **Alcoholic Intoxication:** In case of alcoholic intoxication, consumption of water in which dates have been soaked and mashed brings quick relief.
- **Constipation:** As the dates are mildly laxative in nature they are beneficial in the treatment of constipation. Soak a few dates in water overnight. Crush and form a paste or syrup next morning. Have this daily. The dates provide roughage which stimulates sluggish bowls.
- **General tonic:** Dates being high in sugar and being easily digested are a great store for supplying energy. They act like a tonic in boosting energy levels. Milk in which clean and fresh dates have been boiled is very beneficial and a restorative drink for adults as well as children. The *nicotinic acid* content of dates is an excellent remedy for skin disorders, intestinal disturbances, nervous headaches and insomnia

(sleeplessness). I remember my grandmother making *rice kheer* with 2-3 chopped dates boiling in the milk!
- **Intestinal disorders:** Intestinal disorders or disturbances benefit a lot from the nicotinic acid content of dates. Hence liberal use of dates in your daily diet helps and encourages the growth of friendly bacteria in the intestines and cures intestinal disorders.

More About Dates

The dates can be eaten as a dessert or they can be boiled or stewed in butter. They are also used in fruit salads, cakes and biscuits. Some naturopath suggest the use of date paste as a sweetener in tea, milk, lemon juice etc. For this purpose, puree the dates with water to a fine pulp in a mixer. Store in a bottle in the fridge and use as and when required.

The dates have a sticky surface and hence attract flies, dirt and dust. When buying them make sure that they are packed or covered well. Before use, be sure to wash them thoroughly.

Fig (*Anjeer*)

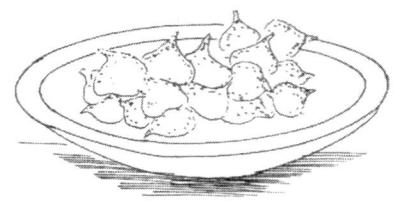

Figs are called a restorative food. It is a pear shaped soft, sweet and pulpy fruit which is a great promoter of health. It is highly recommended for people suffering from general weakness or who are recovering from a prolonged illness. Figs are also known to cool down the body.

The fruit is actually a receptacle with a short stalk and is found in clusters on the trunk and branches of its trees. They can be green, purple or pink or even red when ripe. The fruit being highly perishable is generally sold in the dry form which is highly nutritive as it contains **iron, copper** and other minerals including trace elements like zinc, Vitamin A and a high concentration about 50% - 60% of invert sugar.

The skin being very tough, the dried figs should preferably be soaked in water as then they become easily digestible. However, the water in which they are soaked should also be drunk as a lot of nutrients escape into the water. A decoction of the ripe fruit is used to check leprosy, excessive bleeding during Menstruation, nose bleeding and for expelling intestinal worms. A decoction of the unripe fruit acts as a tonic and gives vitality to the body. It also checks the congestion of liver, leucaemia and problems related to blood.

NATURAL HEALING THROUGH FIGS

- **Asthma:** People suffering from asthma and phlegmatic cough benefit greatly by the consumption of figs. The figs have the property of draining out the phlegm and thus give relief to the patients.

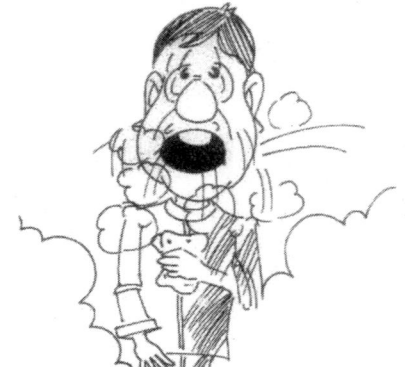

- **Constipation:** As the figs contain a large cellulose content and a thick skin, they are very beneficial in the treatment of constipation. Soak 2-3 dried figs in 1 cup water. Next morning add 1 tablespoon of honey and consume these along with the water in which they were soaked. Continue for at least 1 month. Consumption of fresh figs is also beneficial in curing constipation.
- **Kidney and bladder stones:** Fig consumption is beneficial in these conditions. Boil 6-7 figs in 1 cup of water. Cool and drink daily for at least a month. In case of kidney stones drinking juice of fresh figs frequently is also very beneficial.
- **Piles:** The figs being laxative in nature are a great help and an excellent remedy for piles. Clean 3-4 dried figs well. Wash with warm water and then soak them in 1 cup or 1 glass of water, preferably in an enamel container overnight. Next morning eat these and drink the water also in which they are soaked. Similarly soak 3-4 figs in the morning and have them in the evening. Continue this treatment for at least a month.

As there is no straining at the time of evacuation, piles get cured in due course.

- **Inflammation of spleen:** In this condition, consumption of 2-3 figs along with a cup of curd at least twice a day is very beneficial. This should be continued for a few weeks.
- **Sexual weakness:** Dry figs along with almonds and dry dates roasted in butter are said to be beneficial in cases of sexual weakness.

More About Figs

Figs are generally eaten as a dry fruit. They are also used in the preparation of desserts, Ice creams and cakes. Fresh ripe figs are consumed as a fruit. It is juicy, wholesome and delicious.

Figs should be washed well. They are mostly sold in the dry form. Hence, during handling and transportation attract a lot of dust.

Grapefruit (*Chakotra*)

Grapefruit is a large fruit belonging to the citrus family. It is generally greenish yellow in colour and the juicy flesh inside varies in colour from a pale yellow to pink. The outer skin is usually quite thick. Grapefruit is also called the fruit of paradise as it possesses refreshing and appetising properties.

The fresh fruit has a sharp sub-acid taste but has an alkaline reaction in our systems. It has more or less the same properties as oranges, lemon and sweet lime. It is rich in **vitamin C**, contains some quantity of vitamin A, B1, B2 and P. Fair amounts of calcium and phosphorus are present as well as a small amount of iron is also present.

Grapefruits are of 3 major types:

- White or pink
- Red Star Ruby
- Rio Red

NATURAL HEALING THROUGH GRAPEFRUIT

- **Malaria and feverish colds:** Consumption of grapefruit during feverish colds and Malaria is highly recommended. Grapefruit contains a natural `quinine' which makes it very useful in malaria treatment. Boil half a grapefruit with some water and strain the pulp. Have this 1-2 times a day.
- **Diabetes:** 3 grapefruits taken 3 times a day by a diabetic (one who is not on insulin) will help him to get his sugar under control. People having a tendency to sugar should have 3 grapefruits a day to prevent the development of diabetes. Diabetics should include a liberal amount of grapefruit in their daily diets, but they should along with this also decrease starches, sugars and fats. In the juice form it is recommended that a diabetic consumes ½ a litre of grape juice a day.

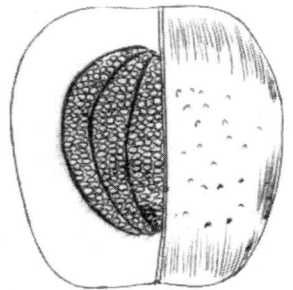

- **Acidity:** The grapefruit like all other citrus fruits has an alkaline reaction in our bodies. Hence consumption of the fresh fruit or its juice is beneficial in the prevention and treatment of acidity and all other ailments caused by too much acid in the digestive system.
- **Constipation:** Consumption of grapefruit helps in relieving constipation as it supplies bulk to facilitate bowel movement.
- **Toning up arteries and lessening the risk of high B.P:** Grape fruits contain a vitamin called vitamin P which helps in the above conditions. Hence regular consumption of the fruit tones up the arteries and reduces the risk of developing high B.P.
- **Stomach disorders:** Grapefruit is a light food and so is good to cure indigestion. It also removes heat from the body and cures stomach irritations. As it has tonic properties it is recommended in cases of biliousness, i.e. in patients with poor digestion.
- **Appetizer:** Grapefruit is an excellent appetizer. It promotes salivary and gastric juice digestion. Hence it is a great health builder and tonic.

More About Grapefruits

Nothing can beat the flavour and succulent goodness of the fresh fruit. Being an appetizer, it is very popular as a breakfast fruit or juice.

It is used in making salads and marmalades which have a tangy refreshing flavour.

Mixed with other fruit or vegetable juices it provides us with a thirst quencher which is very high in vitamins.

Normally a grape fruit is cut into half. Remove the seeds and pith and sprinkle some sugar or brown sugar on it. Chill for a while and enjoy it as a delicious refreshing dessert.

Grapes (*Angoor*)

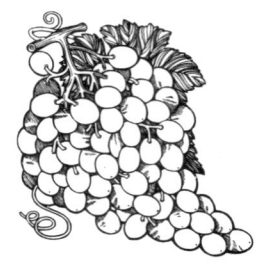

Grapes are one of the oldest cultivated fruits. They are found in bunches on vines and can be green, black or violet, or even reddish in colour. They are oval or round in shape and vary in size. The small ones are seedless whereas the large ones are with 2-3 seeds. It is a delicious fruit which is very nutritious and easily digestible.

Grapes contain a large amount of sugar mainly in the form of glucose. The sugar in the grape gets digested and absorbed very fast and so gives quick heat and energy to the body. Hence grapes are considered nature's great gift to mankind due to its revitalizing and refreshing properties. The grape has an exceptional diuretic value on account of its high content of water and **potassium salts**.

Natural Healing Through Grapes

- **Kidney troubles:** It is a great diuretic and an excellent food remedy in kidney and bladder stones and acute and chronic nephritis, because of its low sodium content.
- **Indigestion and Burning Sensation in the stomach:** Grapes form a light food and so help in overcoming indigestion. They have a soothing effect on excessive secretion of bile and the burning sensation in the stomach.
- **Getting rid of Alcohol:** People trying to give up consumption of alcohol have a great craving. The grapes or its juice provides the purest form of alcohol. Thus if the person consumes grapes or grape juice the craving is controlled. However an exclusive diet of grapes or grape juice is more beneficial and highly recommended during this time.

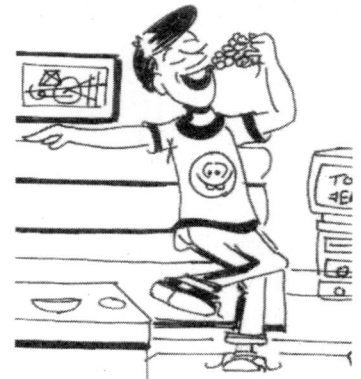

- **Body heat:** Consuming grape juice for some days removes body heat as it cleans and cools the blood.
- **Constipation:** Daily consumption of grapes is highly recommended for people suffering from constipation. The organic acids (malic, citric and tartaric acids) present in grapes in combination with the sugar and cellulose, stimulate the activity of the bowels thus curing constipation. However a minimum of 300-400 gms of grapes or their juice should be taken daily. When fresh grapes are not available soak 10-12 raisins or *kishmish* (dried grapes) in 1 cup of water overnight and consume them the next morning along with the water in which they are soaked for beneficial results.
- **Piles:** As grapes cure constipation, they give relief in cases of piles.
- **Liver disorders:** The malic, citric and tartaric acids found in grapes stimulate the liver and bile secretion. They are therefore beneficial in all liver disorders.
- **Migraine:** Having grape juice in small quantities frequently (a few times daily) brings relief in migraine cases.

- **Anaemia:** Although the iron content in grapes is very little, it is very easily absorbed by the human body. Researchers have found that having 300 ml of grape juice daily can be very beneficial in cases of anaemia.
- **Heart Disease:** Grapes tone up the heart and are beneficial in cardiac pain and palpitations. The disease is controlled effectively if the patient goes on an exclusive grape diet for a few days.
- **Cancer:** Research has shown that grapes contain *ellagin acid*, one of the very highly recommended photo chemicals with a restraining influence on cancer. In the grape cure treatment for cancer, the patient is required to get his body cleansed thoroughly through nature cure treatment. He is asked to fast for 2-3 days on water alone and is also given an enema. On the day the grape cure starts, the patient is given 1-2 glasses of cold water in the morning. After an hour or so, a glass of grape juice is given. Then every 2 hours grape juice is given, 6-7 times in a day. So during the whole day 5-6 litres of grape juice is consumed by the patient. This treatment is known to cure cancer. This

is continued for 1-2 weeks and if found helpful is continued longer. This treatment however should be undertaken only under the guidance and advice of an experienced naturopath. In the nature cure centre of Urulikanchan, near Pune, this treatment is given to patients very successfully.

GRAPES FOR BEAUTY

Mash a few grapes. Apply on face. Leave for 15-20 minutes. Then rinse off for a healthy, glowing and a blemish free complexion.

MORE ABOUT GRAPES

As it is high in sugar people suffering from diabetes should consume them sparingly. It is also made into sherbets and jams and used in salads and desserts. Wine is made from grapes. Grapes do not have a long life and get spoilt very fast.

Guava (*Amrood*)

The Guava tree bears fruit twice a year - in winters and the rainy season. Guava is more beneficial in winters as the guava of the rainy season generally has worms or insects in it.

The guava is a roundish fruit, yellowish or greenish in colour. The flesh of the guava is soft and is generally whitish. Some varieties have a water melon pink flesh. It has a central ball of small, edible but quite hard seeds. The skin of the guava is very thin and the fruit needs only washing and not peeling.

Most of the nutrients and vitamins are present just beneath the skin of the guava, so do not peel it but wash it nicely. Guava is a rich source of vitamin C. It contains a far higher amount of vitamin C than most of the imported and local fruits. It contains **3-6 times more vitamin C than oranges, 10-30 times more than bananas and about 10 times more than papaya.** Most of the vitamin C is concentrated in the skin and the amount of vitamin

C in the fruit reaches the maximum in the green, fully mature fruit and declines as the fruit ripens. They also have an high **iron** content. Regular consumption of the fruit is believed to help reduce and prevent hypertension, high blood pressure and influenza.

Natural Healing Through Guava

- **Stomach disorders:** Guava is excellent for indigestion and flatulence (*gas*). People prone to stomach disorders should eat 250 gms, (about 2 small) guavas a day.
- **Constipation:** The ripe fruit is mildly laxative. It is good to have it for breakfast.
- **Toothache:** The leaves of the guavas are also beneficial. Chewing the tender leaves of a guava tree is good for most of the tooth problems like toothache, swollen gums and infection in the teeth. Boil some leaves in water and gargle with this water to get relief from toothache. It is not a problem to get guava leaves as most of the time the fruit is sold along with a few leaves.

- **Cold:** People prone to cold should consume guava through out winters. This will protect them from cold throughout the year. This is because of the high content of vitamin C present in the guava.

More About Guavas

Guava has a distinctive fragrance. Ripe guavas are good to eat but some prefer a little under-ripe guavas. Guavas are good for the stomach but if eaten in excess may lead to a stomachache.

Guava can be eaten as such or made into a delicious chaat sprinkled with black salt (*kala namak*). Do not drink water after eating the fruit.

Guava jelly is also popular.

Indian Gooseberry (*Amla*)

The **richest source of natural vitamin C,** also called the poor man's source of vitamin C, this small round, 6 lobed fruit is light green in colour. There are two varieties, the wild one which is a smaller fruit and the cultivated one which is a bigger fruit. However both contribute greatly to health and vitality and have great medicinal and beauty powers. It is extensively used in Ayurveda and Tibetan school of medicines.

Experiments have shown that its **vitamin C** is more easily assimilated in our systems than other synthetic forms and it is also **not easily destroyed, not even on boiling.** It also contains calcium, phosphorus, iron and some Vitamin B complex.

Amla is a natural wonder drug. It imparts youthful vigour, cures a whole lot of diseases - diabetes, excessive thirst, anorexia, etc. It acts as a laxative, diuretic and tonic. It also does wonders for your face and hair, tightens up sagging skin and brings lustre to your hair.

Natural Healing Through Amla

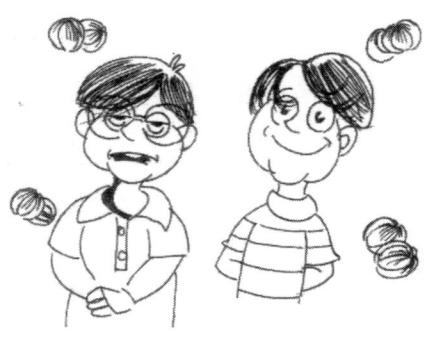

- **Good eyesight:** From the early times our grandmothers have been recommending amla morabba for good eyes and health. It is also recommended for pregnant women. In both the above conditions, it does a world of good due to its high medicinal value.
- **Headache and heaviness in the head:** Grind a few fresh fruit to a fine paste. Apply this on your forehead and rest for a while. You will be surprised to see how fast your problem disappears.
- **Diabetes:** Amla is considered an effective food remedy in diabetes. When fresh fruit is available you can have 1 tablespoon of amla juice mixed with an equal amount of fresh bitter gourd (*karela*) juice in the morning for effective control of diabetes. It will prove very effective in controlling blood sugar and bringing it down.

- **Asthma and Bronchitis:** Drinking a decoction of the seeds of amla, once or twice a day, proves very beneficial in the treatment of all respiratory disorders.
- **Constipation:** Amla is a laxative fruit hence its regular use will help to overcome the problem of habitual constipation. Soak 2-3 dried amlas in water overnight. Next morning, mash them and sieve them. Add a little honey (1-2 teaspoons) and drink this first thing in the morning.
- **Scurvy:** Vitamin C deficiency causes scurvy. Amla is the richest natural source of vitamin C. Consumption of amla in any form will prevent scurvy. When fresh fruit is not available, dried powder can be consumed. As the powder is very sour you can add a little honey to it and have 1-2 teaspoon of amla powder 2-3 times a day with water or milk.
- **Revitalising powder:** Amla is a nourishing and strength giving fruit. It is supposed to posses revitalising powers and also the property to check ageing. It acts as a tonic and increases body resistance against infections.

- **Other ailments:** Consumption of amla fruit in any form - fresh, dried powder, fruit juice form etc. is beneficial in the following problems - gas trouble, flatulence, fevers, vomiting, painful or difficult urination, anaemia, piles, eye disorders, cold, heart and liver problems, skin diseases, nervousness, anxiety, body heat and sexual weakness.

AMLA FOR BEAUTY

Amla is a known hair tonic and a hair nourisher. It also promotes hair pigmentation, which makes the hair dark. Soak dried amla in water overnight. Use this water to rinse hair.

Boil some dried amla pieces in coconut oil for a few minutes. Cool and sieve. Massage hair with this oil regularly for thick and lustrous hair.

In skin problems stop using soap. Instead grind dried amla to a fine powder. Sift it through a very fine strainer and use this to have a bath.

More About Amla

Amla is used in the fresh form to make chutneys, pickles and murabbas.

Amla is very sour and hence excessive consumption may give you a sore throat. Some naturopath are of the opinion that when amla is used for medicinal purposes, meat and sugar should be avoided.

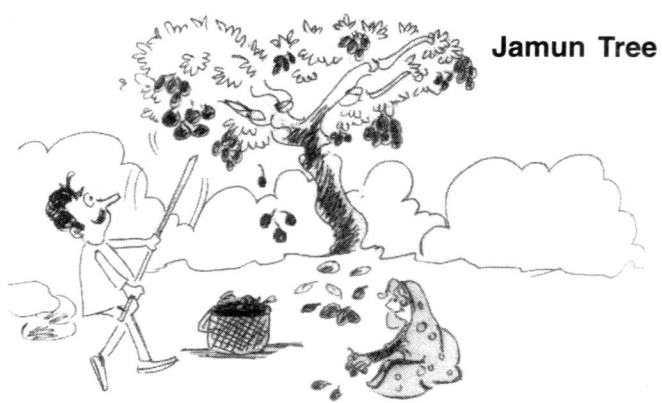

Jamun Tree

Jambul Fruit (*Jamun*)

Jamun is a purplish black oval berry which has a violet flesh inside and one seed that is yellowish green in colour. It is juicy with a sourish, sweet astringent taste.

NATURAL HEALING THROUGH JAMBUL FRUIT

- **Diabetes:** Jamun has the unique position in the fruit kingdom as it is regarded as the most effective and traditional natural medicine for diabetes. The fruit as such, the seeds of the fruit and fruit juice, are all very useful to control the blood and urine sugar. The seeds contain a glucose called *Jamboline* that is said to have the power of checking the conversion of starch into sugar in cases of increased glucose production. The seeds should be dried and powdered. ½ teaspoon of this powder mixed with a little water should be given 2-3 times a day.

- **Piles:** Eating a few jamuns every morning either with salt or with honey proves to be very effective in controlling and curing bleeding piles.
- **Liver problems:** Consumption of ripe jamuns is said to stimulate the liver. Hence they are very beneficial in all liver problems.
- **Varicose veins:** Varicose veins are those blue, ugly swollen veins that can be seen in the legs or on the hands. They come up suddenly and never seem to go away. They may be located anywhere in the body and may be itchy or painful. Consumption of jamuns proves specially beneficial as they contain antioxidants-anthocyanin and ronthocyanidins) which help to strengthen and tone the venous walls so that they do not swell and bleed.

More About Jambul Fruit

Sherbets are also made out of the ripe fruit.

The Jamun has a sour astringent taste. Hence if consumed in excess will cause throat irritation and a sore throat. They may also cause cough and phlegm collection.

Muskmelon (*Kharbooja*)

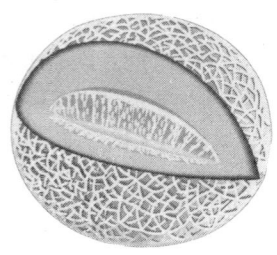

Muskmelon is a delicious fruit, easily available during summers. The hotter it is, the sweeter the melon gets. There are many varieties available but the Lucknow variety with a thin peel and lines on it is very popular.

The flesh of the muskmelon is yellowish red and sometimes yellowish green. It has a lot of seeds which are tasty as well as healthy.

NATURAL HEALING THROUGH MUSKMELON

- **Constipation:** It keeps you away from constipation, which is the root cause of many problems.
- **Jaundice:** It is good for people suffering from jaundice as the toxins are removed through the urine by consuming this high water content fruit.

More About Muskmelon (*Kharbooja*)

Always cool the melon before eating it. Eating too much of this fruit may be harmful as you may get skin eruptions in the form of boils. Too much melon also weakens the intestines and so the person has less resistance towards illnesses, specially cholera during summers.

Lemon (*Niboo*)

Lemon is a very common and easily available fruit. In fact it is called a health fruit as it is beneficial in a lot of ailments. We in India associate it more with vegetables than with fruit as it is sold by the vegetable vendor.

Lemon is oval in shape. It is green in colour when unripe but changes to a lemon yellow colour on ripening. It is sour in taste and it is believed that this sour taste (because of the acids present in lemon juice) is responsible for all the therapeutic value associated with lemon.

Lemon is very rich in citric acid and **vitamin C**, however it also contains minerals like calcium, phosphorus, Iron and some amounts of vitamin A and vitamin B complex.

Lemon is regarded as a great beauty aid in addition to its medicinal value.

Natural Healing Through Lemon

- **Vomiting:** Mix ½ teaspoon lemon juice with ½ teaspoon honey and lick 2-3 times a day. This remedy is very helpful in checking and controlling vomiting.
- **Lowering body heat:** Drinking niboo pani i.e. lemon juice diluted with water and salt-sugar added to taste, lowers body heat. It is not possible to drink pure lemon juice as it is very sour. That is why niboo pani is consumed during summers and a consumption of 3-5 glasses a day is very cooling.
- **Digestive aid:** Lemon is a great appetizer and a promoter of digestion. It stimulates the production of saliva and gastric juice and acts as a good digestive aid. It is also beneficial in gas trouble, controlling nausea, vomiting and curing constipation. Regular intake of lemon juice with 1 teaspoon of honey in a glass of warm water, first thing in the morning proves an effective remedy in constipation.
- **Cough:** Lemon juice has the property of dislodging phlegm. It's consumption pulls out the phlegm and cures cough.

- **Arthritis, Rheumatism, Gout:** Excess acid in the body creates a lot of problems that manifest themselves as swellings, aches and pains such as gout, arthritis, rheumatism etc. To neutralise this acidic condition of the body intake of lemon in sufficient quantities is recommended. The lemon has an alkaline reaction in our bodies and prevents the accumulation of uric acid in the tissues because of which an attack of gout can take place. The ideal way to consume lemon juice is to mix juice of ½ lemon in 1 glass of hot water (as hot as you can drink). Have this 2-3 times a day.
- **Antibacterial:** Lemon juice is a powerful antibacterial. It has been proved by experiments that the bacteria of many diseases such as cholera, diphtheria and typhoid are destroyed by lemon juice. Hence consumption of lemon juice proves beneficial in these diseases. However a regular intake of lemon juice in the form of niboo-pani or juice added to your food could act as a preventive of these diseases.
- **Beneficial to heart:** Lemon is very rich in potassium and hence its consumption is beneficial to the heart.

- **Cold:** Squeeze 1 lemon in a glass of hot water. Add 1-2 teaspoon of honey and 1 teaspoon brandy to it. Have at bedtime. Only lemon juice and honey in hot water can be taken if you do not want to take brandy. This will help you overcome the cold and give you a good night's sleep. It is often said, "A lemon a day keeps the cold away".
- **Diuretic:** Lemon juice being diuretic in nature benefits and gives relief in kidney and bladder disorders.
- **High B.P:** Have 1 cup of butter milk to which 1 teaspoon of lemon juice has been added to bring down your B.P. Have this as frequently as possible.
- **Scurvy:** This is caused by a deficiency of vitamin C. Lemon is also called a poor man's main source of vitamin C as it is very high in vitamin C. It helps cure and prevent scurvy.

LEMON FOR BEAUTY

To give body and shine to your hair, mix together juice of 1 lemon in a mug of cold water. After shampoo, put your head down and pour on wet hair for the final rinse.

Natural Cleanser and Astringent: Dip cotton wool in lemon juice and clean your face regularly with it. This will help cleanse your skin and pores and also help in tightening it. The lemon juice can be left on the face for 15-20 minutes before washing off with water.

Mix some lemon juice with curd, fine oatmeal or besan and mashed carrots (optional) and apply on the face. Leave for 15-20 minutes and then wash off with warm water. This is an excellent skin cleansing mask and should be used on the face and neck at least once a week. However it can also be applied on the arms and other parts of the body.

Marks and Blemishes: Mix equal amounts of lemon juice, coconut oil and sandalwood powder. Make a smooth paste and apply on your face. Let it dry and then wash off. Use this mask everyday for a few days till you see the marks and blemishes disappear from your face.

Soft Feet and Hands: Mix equal amounts of lemon juice and glycerine in a bottle. Apply on feet overnight and preferably wear socks for sometime at least. This will keep your feet soft and cracks on your heels will disappear.

Rub a slice of lemon or apply lemon juice on your elbows regularly. Leave for 20-25 minutes before washing off. The lemon juice will soften your elbows and also lighten them.

Mix little granulated sugar with lemon juice. Gently rub on to your hands till sugar dissolves. Wash off. This makes your hands not only very clean but softens them too.

4-5 tablespoon rose water mixed with 2-3 tablespoon glycerine and 2-3 tablespoon lemon juice and applied on hands and elbows works wonders on them. This mixture can be made and kept in the fridge.

More About Lemon

Lemon juice is highly acidic and sour. Excessive consumption may harm the enamel of the teeth. Excessive consumption is also said to have an adverse effect on the reproductive system.

Mango (*Aam*)

Mango is called the king of fruits and occupies a unique place in the Indian hearts and homes. It's leaves are used for decoration in marriages and other religious functions. Mango is indigenous to India and is considered a valuable food and an excellent home remedy for various ailments.

There are many varieties of mangoes. However the good varieties are the ones that have a thin rind, a small stone and bristleless pulp. Mangoes are said to be heaty, therefore the ideal way of eating them is by first drowning them in cold water for a couple of hours, that is cooling them. Plain water should not be drunk after eating mangoes.

Mango is well known for its medicinal properties both in the ripe and unripe stages. The ripe fruit is very wholesome and excellent source of **vitamin A** and natural sugars. It is fairly rich in **vitamin C.** A mango has 40% Vitamin A and 15 % Vitamin C needed by us in one day. It also contains some thiamin, niacin and riboflavin (vitamin B group). Malic acid, tartaric acid and traces of citric acid are present. The astringency of the fruit can be attributed to the presence of these acids which help in maintaining the alkali reserve of the body. The ripe fruit has a high proportion of carotene which are less in unripe mangoes. However the unripe mango is a rich source of vitamin C and pectin which reduce as the fruit matures.

NATURAL HEALING THROUGH MANGO

- **Acidity:** Milk in combination with mangoes in the form of milk shakes, puddings or mango custard is called the ideal combination as the presence of milk supplies the protein not present in the mango and also controls acidity.
- **Cleaning the body:** Mangoes are said to possess cleansing properties. They cleanse the body by eliminating the toxins present. In fact it is said that when you get boils on consumption of mangoes it is a sign that the toxins are being expelled in the form of these skin eruptions.

- **Eye problems:** Mangoes are very rich in vitamin A and so their liberal consumption is very beneficial in various eye disorders. Night blindness, very common in undernourished children, is caused due to vitamin A deficiency. These patients benefit greatly by liberal consumption of mangoes.
- **Digestive and Liver problems:** Suck or eat a mango and then drink a glass of milk after it for a few days, to get maximum benefit in liver and digestive disorders.
- **Rickets:** Unripe mango consumption is very beneficial in the treatment of rickets. Mix 1 teaspoon of dried unripe mango powder (*amchoor*) with an equal amount of honey and have it at least twice a day for sometime.
- **Weight gain:** Mango is a very nourishing fruit. It is rich in sugar and hence the consumption of mangoes is beneficial for people who are underweight. In fact a combination of mango and milk taken 3-4 times a day is highly recommended for weight gain. Milk has no sugar and mango has no protein, whereas mango is rich in sugar and milk in protein. Therefore they compliment each other very well.

- **Blood disorders and Scurvy:** The unripe mango is very rich in vitamin C. It helps in the formation of blood cells and increases resistance of the body against various diseases such as TB, anaemia, dysentery etc. Scurvy which is caused due to vitamin C deficiency can be overcome by daily consumption of unripe mangoes or by consuming *amchoor* - a common spice made from raw mangoes and used for cooking in all Indian households.
- **Heat Stroke:** A drink called *panna* made from unripe mangoes is a very effective remedy for heat stroke. Cook 3-4 unripe mangoes with some water till soft and tender. Peel the mangoes. Mash and then strain. To this sieved water, either add jaggery (*gur*) or sugar and salt to taste. Mix well. Put some of this mixture in a glass and add some cold water to it and have it as a drink. Some mint leaves paste can also be added to the above drink for a better flavour and cooling effect. In places that have a severe summer, generally all Indian households, consume *panna* through out summer as a preventive for heat exhaustion and heat stroke.

More About Mango

Ripe mango is the king of fruits and enjoys the highest position as a fruit or a dessert. Jams, jelly, squash, crush etc. are also prepared from ripe mangoes.

Unripe mangoes are used for making amchoor, pickles, chutneys, curries and sherbets.

People suffering from skin diseases and stomach ulcers are advised to avoid mangoes. If you have consumed too many mangoes it is advisable to consume a handful of Jamun as an antidote or drink an infusion of cumin *(jeera)* to felicitate the digestion of mangoes. Raw mango is sour and therefore excessive consumption may lead to throat irritation or sore throat. It can also lead to indigestion and dysentery. Water should never be drunk over mangoes as it causes irritation.

Consuming too many ripe mangoes causes dysentery, eye infection and fever. People also get boils due to excessive mango intake.

Mulberry (*Shahtoot*)

The mulberry tree is quite big and dense. The fruit has various sizes, ranging from ½" to 2-3" in length. The fruit is greenish or dark reddish in colour.

NATURAL HEALING THROUGH MULBERRY

- **Enhances appetite**: During fever it also helps in digestion and thus enhances appetite.
- **Ulcers in the mouth:** The sherbet of this fruit is very beneficial for people having ulcers (*chhale*) in the mouth and throat.
- **Fever:** It is an excellent thirst quencher. Its sherbet is very soothing during summers. It is very cooling for patients suffering from fever.

MORE ABOUT MULBERRY

Check for worms before eating, which may be present in the fruit. In summers it is beneficial to have the fruit 2-3 hours after lunch. It helps overcome the heat produced in the body and also cleanses the blood.

Orange (*Santra*)

When we think of consuming vitamin C in its natural form, the fruit that comes to our minds is the good old orange. Orange belongs to the citrus family. It is yellow-green, orange-yellow to bright orange in colour and round in shape. Skin is somewhat rough and thick and is loose so that it can be easily removed by hand. Seeds are many.

Orange is a rich source of vitamin C. Our daily requirement of vitamin C is met by drinking approximately 200 ml (1 cup) of orange juice daily. As the vitamin C in orange is protected by the presence of citric acid, it is not easily destroyed. The rich membranes surrounding the sections of oranges and the fruit itself is a very rich source of **calcium** practically superior to any other fruit. However this fact is not very well known by people who think only of vitamin C when they think of oranges. In addition oranges also contain copper, sulphur, potassium, sodium, iron, chlorine, vitamin A and vitamin B. Thus consuming oranges is very beneficial for our health.

Natural Healing Through Orange

- **Constipation:** Consuming 3-4 oranges a day or drinking orange juice daily will take care of this problem. The best way to have oranges for this problem is at breakfast and before retiring at night.
- **Appetizer:** Oranges are great appetizers and that is why it is seen that orange juice is included in breakfast all over the world. It is delicious, nourishing and contains readily assimilable sugar that can be readily absorbed in our blood to provide us with energy for immediate use.
- **Asthma and other bronchial troubles:** Orange juice mixed with a pinch of salt and 1 tablespoon honey if drunk regularly loosens the collected phlegm, thus benefiting the patient greatly.
- **Digestive aid:** Oranges are very useful and act as a digestive aid by creating a condition in the intestines which are conducive to the development of friendly bacteria.
- **Heart disease:** Orange juice sweetened with honey is a great nourishing and energy giving food. It is therefore recommended for heart patients particularly when one is on a liquid diet. It is also a

good remedy against the thickening of arterial walls.

- **Bones and Teeth:** Oranges being a rich source of calcium which is readily absorbed by our bodies due to the presence of vitamin C in the fruit is a great builder of teeth and bones and also helps in warding of their diseases like cavities and pyorrhoea etc.
- **Resistance of the body:** Oranges or orange juice although acidic in taste has an alkaline reaction in our bodies. After being metabolised it leaves an alkaline residue and thus improves the vital resistance of the body which enables us to fight infections, colds, fevers etc. In addition having oranges or orange juice is beneficial for the eyes, in painful inflammation of joints, rheumatism, kidney and bladder stones and different types of cysts and tumours. It also strengthens the bones and increases muscle tone and is good for the nervous system.

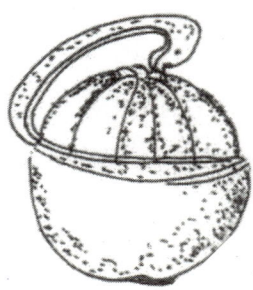
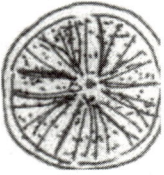

Orange For Beauty

A good moisturising and toning mask for dry skin. Mix together 1 tablespoon orange juice with ½ tablespoon honey and apply on the face. Let it dry for 15-20 minutes and then wash off. You can also add 1 teaspoon of fullers earth *(multani mitti)* to it. Increase the amount of honey and orange juice to get a smooth paste.

Apply fresh orange peel paste on the corn. They will soften in a short time.

Applying plain fresh orange juice on your face makes your complexion rosy.

More About Orange

Orange/orange juice is used as a table fruit and a breakfast drink. It is used in the preparation of various sauces, marmalades, sherbets, desserts and salads. Oil from it's skin is used in perfumes. The peel is also used in herbal cosmetics.

Papaya (*Papita*)

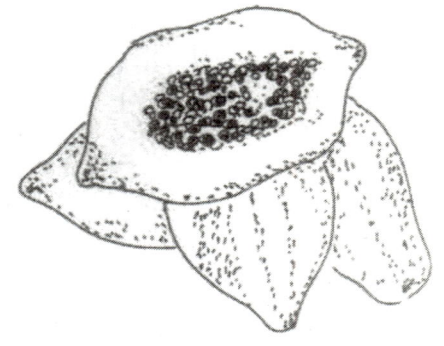

Papaya is a well known, cheap and easily available sweet fruit. It has the distinction of one of the most rapidly growing plants. Within a year the tree bears fruit. The ripe fruit is oval or roundish in shape and varies in colour from yellow to orangish. It has a central hollow cavity which has numerous small black seeds. However seedless varieties are also available now.

The ripe papaya is a wholesome fruit. It is high in **vitamin C** and ½ a papaya fulfils 150% of our daily requirement of vitamin C. The fresh fruit is also a source of natural sugars, **vitamin A** and an enzyme called papain which is similar to pepsin found in our stomachs. Papain prevents improper protein breakdown in the system thus preventing many allergies and stomach ailments.

NATURAL HEALING THROUGH PAPAYA

- **Cancer:** Papaya contains different types of enzymes due to which it is said to be effective in the treatment of cancer. After treatment with antibiotics, the use of papaya or papaya juice hastens the restoration of the friendly symbiotic bacteria in the alimentary canal which had been destroyed by the use of powerful drugs.
- **Constipation:** Daily consumption of papaya is a sure way of getting rid of constipation. In addition, its regular consumption also cures bleeding piles, chronic dysentery and hyperacidity.
- **Digestion:** Papaya is a very easily digested fruit and it also helps in the digestion of other foods.
- **Enlargement of spleen:** Skin a ripe fruit and cut into small pieces. Immerse in vinegar for a week. Consume approx. 2-3 tablespoon of this preserved fruit along with your meals at least 2-3 times a day.

- **Increasing milk in nursing mothers:** Eating cooked unripe fruit, green papaya as a vegetable, frequently helps in increasing the milk in young nursing mothers.
- **Liver and Spleen inflammation:** Take a large slice of papaya with 1 teaspoon of honey every day to control the inflammation of spleen and liver. Avoiding fats, starches, sugar will give better results.
- **Rejuvenating property:** Papaya is said to have rejuvenating properties and thus can control ageing. Papaya cleanses the body and acts as an excellent tonic and energy giving food.
- **Throat disorders:** Inflamed tonsils, diptheria and other throat disorders benefit greatly by the application of fresh juice of raw papaya mixed with some honey. It is effective in dissolving the membrane and preventing infection from spreading.
- **Virility:** Consumption of ripe papaya increases virility. It is also very beneficial for the heart. It alleviates insanity and being diuretic in nature does a lot of good in urinary disorders. Ayurveda experts regard papain as a remedy for abdominal disorders and in regulating and securing proper menstruation flow.

Papaya For Beauty

Papaya makes an excellent nourishing and rejuvenating mask. Mash a piece of ripe papaya and apply on the face and neck. Leave for 15-20 minutes and then wash off. Papaya contains enzymes which soften and remove dead cell bringing a lustre to the face. It also helps in curing pimples. In addition to this, it also prevents wrinkles.

Grate some raw papaya. Squeeze out the juice. Apply juice regularly on face to get rid of all the blemishes.

More About Papaya

Ripe papaya is eaten as a breakfast fruit. Unripe papaya is cooked as a vegetable. Ripe papaya is also used to make jams, cold drinks and fruit salads. Papain which is obtained from the latex of the plant is used in medicine, pharmacy and for tenderizing of meat (meat tenderiser). The enzyme is also included in chewing gums and some foods specially prepared for children.

Pineapple (*Ananas*)

Pineapple is an extremely popular and a delicious juicy fruit. It is oblong and looks like a pine-cone and hence the name pineapple.

The fresh fruit is high in **vitamin A**, **vitamin C** while the B vitamins - thiamin, riboflavin, niacin and vitamin E are present in small quantities. Pineapples are rich in **minerals as they contain phosphorus, calcium, magnesium, iron and copper.**

NATURAL HEALING THROUGH PINEAPPLE

Cancer: Pineapples have an alkaline reaction in our bodies. It is the most essential foodstuff in the cancer diet. In fact it is included in the menu everyday. It is said that if you go on an exclusive pineapple diet for one week every few months you will never get cancer. It is said to be a preventive against cancer.

Digestive: Pineapple or pineapple juice has virtually the same digestive and medicinal properties as papaya juice. It also contains a protein digesting enzyme called Bromelin. This enzyme also has a particular action on casein, the principal protein in milk. It breaks down the protein for easy assimilation by our bodies. Hence pineapple acts as a great digestive aid.

Pineapple For Beauty

A cuticle softening and nourishing cream can be made very easily at home. Mix together 4 tablespoon pineapple juice, 1 teaspoon cider vinegar and 4 tablespoon egg yolk. Mix every thing well and massage nails and cuticles with it. Leave it on for 20-25 minutes. Then wash off.

More About Pineapple

It is eaten as a table fruit and probably it is one fruit which is extensively used in its canned form. It is not as nutritious as the fresh fruit but even in the canned form, it is still rich in vitamin A, calcium and phosphorous.

The pineapple is a little sour in taste. Hence excessive consumption may lead to a sore throat or throat irritation. It also makes your mouth rough and irritated.

Pomegranate (*Anar*)

Pomegranate, also called a **heart's tonic** is a fairly large fruit (the size of a large orange and has a smooth leathery skin. It ranges in colour from brownish yellow to red to deep maroon. Inside it is divided into several cells containing numerous angular elongated or round seeds. They are protected or surrounded by transparent reddish pulp which is very juicy and has a delicious sub-acid flavour.

Pomegranate is considered auspicious by the Chinese and they believe that it wards off evil.

Pomegranate is delicious having a refreshing and soothing taste. The juice is a great thirst quencher and is held in high esteem for it's taste as well as it's medicinal properties. In fact it has been described as a heart tonic.

Natural Healing Through Pomegranate

- **Improving blood and anaemia:** Drinking pomegranate juice frequently is very beneficial in anaemia and in improving the quality of blood. Add some powdered cinnamon (*dalchini*) and cloves (*laung*) to the juice.
- A combination of pomegranate juice mixed with some honey and cinnamon powder is very beneficial and also very delicious.
- **Diarrhoea and dysentery:** Pomegranate is said to be constipating, hence it is useful in the control of diarrhoea and dysentery.

  For controlling **diarrhoea**, drinking 40-50 ml (¼ cup) of fresh juice proves to be very effective.

  In the case of **dysentery**, powder the outer (rind) skin finely. Mix 1 teaspoon of skin (rind) powder with ¼ teaspoon nutmeg powder (grated *jaiphal*) and 1 teaspoon of pure ghee. Mix well and have at least 2-3 times daily till the condition improves.
- **Asthma, cough:** Pomegranate juice is extremely beneficial in asthma

and cough. Mix together equal quantities of pomegranate juice, fresh ginger juice and honey. Take 1-2 tablespoon of this mixture 2-3 times a day for quick and speedy relief. A cold drink or juice of ripe fruit is also highly recommended.

- **Burning Sensation during Urination and Sexual Weakness** - Grind 2-3 teaspoon dried pomegranate seeds and 1-2 times a day with milk for relief.

More About Pomegranate

It is widely used as a table fruit and in salads. Sherbets and cooling drinks are made from the fruit and are very valuable in relieving thirst in feverish conditions. Pomegranates are also used to make wine. Perhaps the most romantic use of the fruit is made in a Turkish wedding. The bride throws a pomegranate to the ground and the seeds that spill out are counted in the belief that their number equals the number of children she will bear.

Plums (*Aloo Bukhara*)

It is a soft round smooth-skinned sweet fruit with sweet reddish flesh and a flattish pointed stone. Plums are high in carbohydrates, low in fat and low in calories. Plums are an excellent source of vitamin A, calcium, magnesium, iron, potassium and fibre. They are free of sodium and cholesterol. Like all fruits, plums contain a substantial amount of vitamin C. A prune is a dried plum. Chutneys and squashes are made from plums.

NATURAL HEALING THROUGH PLUMS

- **Diarrhoea**: When one gets loose motions due to stomach upset and fever, plums control diarrhoea. The benefit of eating plums during diarrhoea is that they do not lead to constipation.
- **Jaundice:** Plums are beneficial for jaundice patients.
- **Increase appetite:** The consumption of plums increases appetite and helps in the digestion of food.

Peaches (*Aadu*)

It is a round juicy fruit with a hairy yellowish-red skin and a rough stone which has a kernel in it. The flesh is soft, yellowish with a hint of red in it. It is a little sour and is a good source of **vitamin C.**

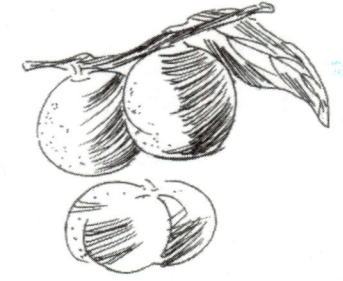

NATURAL HEALING THROUGH PEACHES

- **Teeth and gums:** Consuming peaches strengthens the teeth and gums.

MORE ABOUT PEACHES

Peaches should be eaten when fully ripe. The under-ripe fruit is sour and may hurt the throat and lead to a cough. Also the fine hair being hard on the under-ripe fruit may give rise to throat problems.

Strawberries

It is a delicious pinkinsh fruit with a sweet and sour taste. It has a spotted skin. It has very tiny hair on the skin.

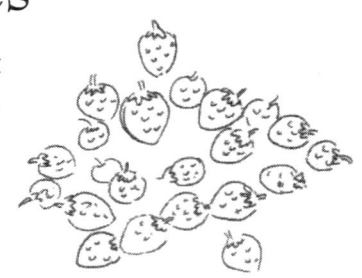

NATURAL HEALING THROUGH STRAWBERRIES

- Strawberries contain a lot of **vitamin C** and **iron**. So it is good for iron deficiency diseases like anaemia.

MORE ABOUT STRAWBERRIES

The allergic reaction that the eating of strawberries can cause is usually caused by the tiny hair on the fruit. There is a good chance that the strawberries will not irritate if you rinse them with hot water before eating. They have to be eaten within one or two days because they are picked when they are ripe. Strawberries whiten the teeth.

Sweet Lime (*Mosambi*)

We are all familiar with sweet lime or *Mosambi* as it is generally called. It is always given to sick people and children for nourishment. Sweet Lime is a delicious and a very popular fruit with a thin rind. It possesses invaluable nutrients. It is very rich in **vitamin C** and **vitamin A.** It also contains **calcium** and **iron.** Mosambi juice increases vitality and resistance to illness. Mosambi or Mosambi juice has no equal and is indispensable in illness.

NATURAL HEALING THROUGH SWEET LIME

- **Acidity:** The ripe fruit has an alkaline reaction in our bodies. It is therefore highly recommended in cases of acidity and windiness. The fruit is an excellent appetiser & quickly normalises the digestive process.
- **Fever:** Mosambi or its juice is easily digested. It quenches thirst, is cooling and highly nourishing. It is therefore an ideal food during sickness when other food is not permitted.

- **Constipation:** The fibrous element of the fruit proves beneficial in overcoming the problem of constipation. It is recommended to eat the fruit as such and not only have its juice when suffering from constipation.
- **Blood purifying:** Mosambi is said to be a blood purifier and that is one of the reasons why it is recommended in all illnesses. Besides being nourishing, it is also said to promote vitality.
- It is also beneficial in vomiting, dehydration and cough.

MORE ABOUT SWEET LIME

Besides being enjoyed as a fruit as such, it is used for salads, desserts, jams and cold drinks.

People prone to colds i.e. those who get cold very often should warm the juice a little before consuming and should consume the fruit at room temperature.

Watermelon (*Tarbuz*)

It is a large fruit, the size of a football. It is either round or oval, deep green in colour or light green streaked with dark green. A thick ring of white flesh surrounds the red fleshy or pulpy part in which numerous flat black seeds are embedded.

NATURAL HEALING THROUGH WATERMELON

- **Anaemia:** The seeds of watermelon are high in iron. Chewing or eating the seeds will be highly effective for people suffering from Anaemia.
- **Constipation:** Watermelon is mildly laxative in nature. Regular consumption of the fruit takes care of any constipation that you might be suffering. 2 medium sized bowls of the fruit should be had daily.
- **Depression:** Watermelon consumption on a regular basis benefits people who are suffering from depression or who are prone to depression.

- **Flow of urine:** The fruit contains a large amount of water. This felicitates the free and easy flow of urine and is also very beneficial in kidney problems and the urinary tract infections. However people with a bladder problem and who cannot control urination, should avoid it.
- **High B.P:** Watermelon is high in potassium but very low in sodium and hence helps in lowering high B.P.
- **Painful Menstruation:** Chop the white ring of pulp under the outer skin and outside the red pulp into pieces. Add little water and churn in the mixer. Sieve. Have this juice every morning for a month daily. You will find that your periods become absolutely painless. However if the pain persists, continue for some more time or start having it twice a day.
- **Weight reduction:** The watermelon is an ideal fruit for people wanting to lose weight. It contains a large amount of water and is very low in its calorie content. Consuming watermelon once or twice a day fills you up and although your stomach is full you have consumed very few calories and hence it aids in weight reduction.

- Watermelon consumption is also helpful in arthritis, indigestion and mouth and throat diseases. The juice of the ripe fruit helps in dissolving kidney and bladder stones.
- The seeds roasted and ground make a good emulsion for inflammation of urinary tract. Eating the seeds reduces high B.P and inflammation of the prostate gland.
- There is no other fruit or fruit juice which is as cooling and a great thirst quencher as watermelon. Hence its consumption specially during the summer months is very satisfying.

More About Watermelon

Ripe watermelon is eaten popularly as a table fruit. It is also made into sorbets, salads and its juice served as a cold refreshing drink.

The small young unripe watermelons are cooked like a vegetable, made into bharta or a delicious raita.

The white pulp of the ripe watermelon is also cooked as a vegetable (sweet and sour) and is extremely popular in Rajasthan.

It is advisable not to consume watermelon during monsoons. Never drink milk after having watermelon as it may cause a stomach upset.

People who are thin, weak and have excessive wind problem should avoid watermelon.

Walnut (*Akhrot*)

The walnut looks like a human brain and incidentally it is believed that this fruit enhances the brain power.

Walnuts are of 2 types - one with a soft skin known as '*Kagzi*' and the other one is with a hard skin. Much of the carved woodwork for which Kashmir is famous uses walnut wood.

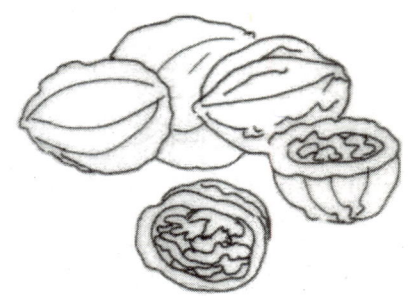

NATURAL HEALING THROUGH WALNUT

- **Stones:** Grind walnut kernels to a powder. Have 1 teaspoon of walnut powder, morning and evening to get rid of stones through the urine.
- **Bed wetting:** Give 2 walnuts and 10-12 raisins (*kishmish*) for 15-20 days to the child just before going to bed, to cure the habit of bed-wetting in children.

- **Vigour:** It imparts vigour and removes impotency.

Walnut For Beauty:

To remove tan and improve a tanned complexion, mix walnut powder with a few drops of vinegar. Apply on the face. Scrub and wash off after 15-20 minutes.

For a good scrub, mix walnut powder with a little rose water and scrub on the face in the upward direction with circular movements to remove dead cells and rejuvenate the skin.

More About Walnuts

Avoid buying walnuts in plastic packets if possible. Always taste walnuts before using them. Old, bitter and rancid walnuts will spoil any dish they are added to.

If keeping walnuts for a long time, store them in the freezer to prevent their high oil content becoming rancid.

Important Points to Remember About Fruits

- The fruit should always be fresh and clean. Overripe fruits should not be eaten. When the fruit starts getting over ripe, it starts losing it's nutritive value.
- Wash fruits very well because they are generally sprayed very heavily with insecticides and other harmful sprays.
- Do not peel fruits which can be had with the peel such as guavas, apples, pears etc.
- Drink fruit juice immediately. On keeping the juice, the vitamin C reduces. Similarly fruits should not be cut and kept in the fridge. They should be consumed as soon as they are cut.
- Fruits should not be consumed with meals. Have them at least 30 minutes before the meals or 2-3 hours after the meals. The digestion time of the two varies greatly.
- Never eat a spoilt fruit. When the fruit goes bad, it can never be good for your body. It might harm you in the bargain.

Index

A

Acidity 30, 44, 70, 91
Alcoholic Intoxication 36, 47
Allergies 24
Anaemia 9, 12, 17, 24, 49, 86, 93
Antibacterial 65
Arthritis, Rheumatism, Gout 12, 25, 65
Asthma 39, 56, 76, 86

B

Bed wetting 97
Blood disorders 72, 92
Blood and anaemia-Improvement 86
Blood Pressure-High 12, 66, 94
B.P-Toning up arteries and lessening the risk 44
Body heat 48, 64
Bones 77
Brain tonic 16
Burns and wounds 25

C

Cancer 16, 25, 30, 49, 80, 83
Cataract 17
Cholera 31
Cold 53, 66
Constipation 9, 13, 16, 25, 36, 40, 44, 48, 52, 56, 61, 76, 80, 92, 93
Cough 13, 64

D

Depression 24, 93
Diabetes 26, 43, 55, 59
Diarrhoea 13, 26, 86, 88
Digestive aid 64, 76, 80, 83
Digestive problems 21, 47, 71
Diuretic 66
Dry Cough 31
Dysentery 22, 26, 86

E

Eye problems 13, 71
Eyesight-Good 55

F

Fever 9, 74, 91

Feet and Hands-Soft 67

H

Headache and heaviness in the head 55
Heart Disease 12, 49, 65, 76
Heart - Weak 35
Heat Stroke 72

I

Increase appetite 88
Increasing milk in nursing mothers 81
Intestinal disorders 37
Intestine-Worms 32

J

Jaundice 61, 88

K

Kidney and bladder stones 40
Kidney and liver disorders 17
Kidney troubles 47

L

Liver and Spleen inflammation 81
Liver problems 21, 48, 60

M

Malaria and feverish colds 43
Malnutrition 21
Marks and Blemishes 67
Menstruation-Painful 94
Migraine 48
Milk for Babies 18
Mouth Ulcer 31, 74

N

Nerve Tonic 13

P

Pain in Hips 31
Piles 26, 31, 40, 48, 60

R

Rejuvenating property 81
Resistance of the body 77
Revitalising powder 56
Rickets 71

S

Scurvy 56, 66, 72
Sexual Weakness 18, 35, 41, 87
Spleen-Enlargement 80
Spleen-Inflammation 41, 81
Stomach disorders 44, 52
Stomach Ulcers 32
Stones 97

T

Teeth and gums 77, 89
Teeth-Protector 14
Teething problems in children 35
Throat disorders 81
Tonic 18
Toothache 52

U

Ulcers 26
Urinary Trouble 32, 87, 94

V

Varicose veins 60
Vigour 98
Virility 81
Vomiting 64

W

Weight gain 71
Weight reduction 94

BEST SELLERS IN QUICK & EASY SERIES

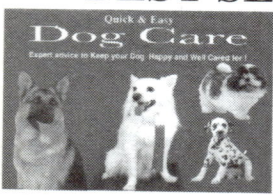
Dog Care

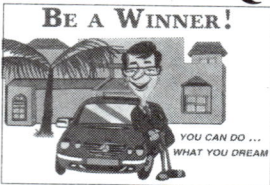
Be A Winner!

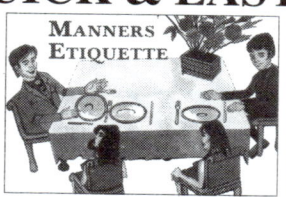
Manners & Etiquette

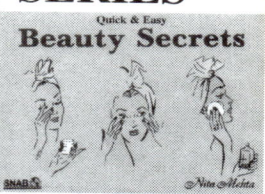
Beauty Secrets

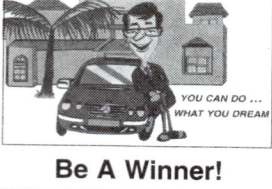
Home Gardening

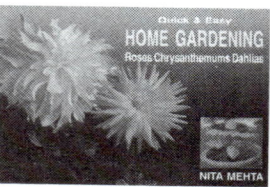
Home Gardening
Roses Chrysanthemums Dahlias

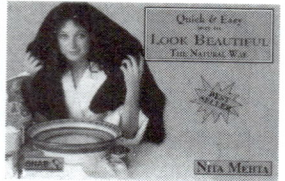
Look Beautiful

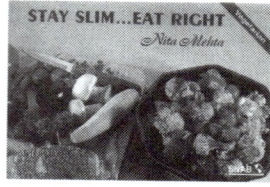
Stay Slim...Eat Right

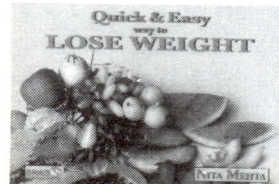
LOSE WEIGHT

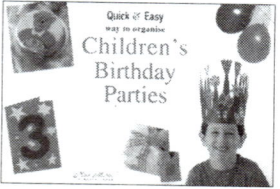
Children's Birthday Parties

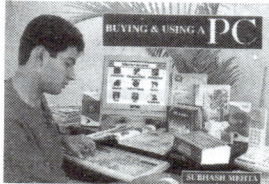
Buying & Using A PC